50 THINGS TO KNOW ABOUT BECOMING A PHYSICIAN ASSISTANT

A Guide to Success in PA Field

I0492611

Elizabeth Maselli

Cover designed by: Ivana Stamenkovic
Cover Image: https://pixabay.com/photos/doctor-stethoscope-medical-2860504/

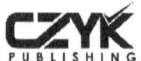

CZYK Publishing Since 2011.

50 Things to Know
Lock Haven, PA
All rights reserved.
ISBN: 9798694002431

50 THINGS TO KNOW ABOUT KNOW ABOUT BECOMING A PHYSICIAN ASSISTANT

50 THINGS TO KNOW BOOK SERIES REVIEWS FROM READERS

I recently downloaded a couple of books from this series to read over the weekend thinking I would read just one or two. However, I so loved the books that I read all the six books I had downloaded in one go and ended up downloading a few more today. Written by different authors, the books offer practical advice on how you can perform or achieve certain goals in life, which in this case is how to have a better life.

The information is simple to digest and learn from, and is incredibly useful. There are also resources listed at the end of the book that you can use to get more information.

50 Things To Know To Have A Better Life: Self-Improvement Made Easy!

Author Dannii Cohen

This book is very helpful and provides simple tips on how to improve your everyday life. I found it to be useful in improving my overall attitude.

50 Things to Know For Your Mindfulness & Meditation Journey
Author Nina Edmondso

Quick read with 50 short and easy tips for what to think about before starting to homeschool.

50 Things to Know About Getting Started with Homeschool by Author Amanda Walton

I really enjoyed the voice of the narrator, she speaks in a soothing tone. The book is a really great reminder of things we might have known we could do during stressful times, but forgot over the years.

Author HarmonyHawaii

There is so much waste in our society today. Everyone should be forced to read this book. I know I am passing it on to my family.

50 Things to Know to Downsize Your Life: How To Downsize, Organize, And Get Back to Basics

Author Lisa Rusczyk Ed. D.

Great book to get you motivated and understand why you may be losing motivation. Great for that person who wants to start getting healthy, or just for you when you need motivation while having an established workout routine.

50 Things To Know To Stick With A Workout: Motivational Tips To Start The New You Today

Author Sarah Hughes

BOOK DESCRIPTION

Did you just get into PA school and want to know what to expect? Are you new to the profession and want to know how to tackle your first few years? Have you been doing this for awhile and need a pick-me-up? If you answered yes to any of these questions then this book is for you...

50 Things to Know about Becoming a Physician Assistant by Elizabeth Maselli offers an approach to show you the tips and tricks of what to expect no matter what stage you are in. Whether you are just starting to consider this field of medicine or have been doing this for several years, this book will provide guidance on how to survive school and your first years in practice, as well as advice for those seasoned Physician Assistants. From surviving your pharmacology courses to finding ways to capture all the important moments in your career, this book will enlighten you on what this amazing profession is all about! We have been given the chance to save lives and to make a difference to thousands of people. You do not want to miss a single step along the way, so grab your copy today! You'll be glad you did.

TABLE OF CONTENTS

DEDICATION

This book is dedicated to my parents, Richard and Laura Bubbico, for teaching me the importance of education.

ABOUT THE AUTHOR

Elizabeth Maselli is a Physician Assistant and freelance writer who lives in Fairfield, CT with her newlywed husband, Don. Elizabeth loves to write, read the bible, and knit. She was bit by the travel bug early on and loves to travel outside of the country at least once a year. She has a successful career in surgery, working both in the clinical and administrative world.

INTRODUCTION

The good physician treats the disease; the great physician treats the patient who has the disease.

-William Osler

This book has been divided into three sections: PA School, The New PA, and The Experienced PA. Each section provides tips and insight on what it is like to be a physician assistant in that stage of life. Although I practice medicine within the specialty of surgery, this book has been written to pertain to all specialties in hopes to have a broader impact for our profession.

PA SCHOOL

1. THEY'VE CHOSEN YOU FOR A REASON

Here is a little insider secret: everyone in your program actually wants you to succeed. They are not there to weed out the weak or to push you so hard that you are unable to graduate. If you fail out or do not pass your boards, it actually looks bad on the program. If you are one of the few people to be blessed enough to be accepted into a PA program, it is because they see the qualities of a successful PA in you. Once you are in, they will try their hardest to get you to graduate and pass your boards. Of course, you have to put in the work, but the program is for you and not against you. Use every resource you can during your didactic training to further your education. Work hard from the very first day until the day you graduate.

2. YOU GET OUT WHAT YOU PUT IN

There is no doubt about it. PA school, no matter what program you attend, is a ton of hard work. There is no skirting around the subject matters. You cannot send someone else to take notes for you, to write your papers, or to take your tests. At the end of the program, you and only you have to take your boards. I have found throughout my career of precepting, teaching and practicing as a PA that the more you put into it, the more you get out of it. The students who spend the extra time with their professors, who study in groups to get others feedback and who put in the sweat and tears are the most successful individuals in the real world. Do not sell yourself short. You are here for a reason. And although you have your entire career to master your specialty, now is the time to absorb as much information as possible. You will be shocked at when and where you use it.

3. COME PREPARED FOR PIMPING

Here is where all of the hard work from tip #2 pays off. There is such a thing as what we call "pimping" in medicine. If you are not familiar with the term it is when a doctor or other practitioner asks you multiple questions rapid fire method on a particular subject matter. It happens most often when you are presenting a patient on your clinical rotations or when you are presenting at a M&M (mortality and morbidity) conference. The best way to be prepared for this is two-fold. First, study as hard as you can in your didactic year. Second, review the subject matter prior to your presentation and write key notes on a card. Before presenting your patient review those notes so they are fresh in your mind, but keep that notecard close by in case you need to reference it. What I have found to be true is the more accurate answers you have right the first time, the less you are "pimped" because the practitioner knows that you know your stuff. They typically only ask questions they know the answers to and we all tend to use the same type of questions. So as time goes on it will be easy for you to prepare. If you do not know the answer, simply say "I don't know but I will look it up and get back to you". This goes a long way and shows you are taking ownership. Sometimes they are kind enough to provide the correct answer for you. Don't forget to keep an extra index card in your pocket to write these answers down.

4.   EVERY DRUG KNOWN TO MAN

I used to joke with my classmates that we deserved a bachelor's degree in a foreign language just for learning all of the names of the medications during pharmacology class (not to mention all of the medical terminology). There are so many medications and such little time. Thankfully, the most common medications are ones we have typically come into contact with during our civilian lives. So here is what you need to know: pharmacology gets easier. Break it down into subsections of types of medications (anti-fungals, NSAIDS, antibiotics). Memorize as many as you can, paying special attention to the most common ones. Remember, common things happen commonly. In other words, you will use the same medications over and over. Learn those first to boost your confidence, and then tackle the harder medications.

Keep in mind you will see all different types of medications on your boards. So please do not think I am saying memorize the common ones and forget the rest. Like the rest of the other classes you will take, you will need to memorize as much as possible.

5.   YOUR SPECIALTY WILL MAKE ITSELF KNOWN

I was invited to give a talk to first year students at a brand-new PA program a few years back. After I was introduced, my opening remark came in the form of two questions to the entire student body. How many people in this room know exactly what specialty they want to enter when they graduate? How many people have no idea what you want to do when you enter the real world? The results were split down the middle. Some students come into PA school knowing exactly what they wanted to do, others come with a few grand ideas of where they wanted to be but no final decision, and the rest had not a single clue. The best piece of advice I can give is take a deep breath. It's okay to have any of those three answers. Just know that during your clinical year, your specialty will likely make itself known to you. It may be one day when you come home and instead of feeling exhausted, you feel exhilarated. It may be from a positive patient interaction you had that day that made you feel at home. Or it may be that you hated every other rotation but this one. However it happens, don't feel like you need to have it all mapped out on the first day. This program is a long journey, and you have time to figure it out.

6. CHANGE IS IN THE AIR

One of the things I know for sure is that PA school changes you. It is impossible to go through such a rewarding, sacrificial time without some serious internal changes. You realize you're stronger and smarter than you think. One of the most impactful life changes I noticed was that the veil was torn. The more educated I became during my didactic year, the more I started to diagnose strangers on the street just by looking at them. I would be sitting on a subway and before I knew it, I was diagnosing the elderly man sitting next to me with Rheumatoid Arthritis just by the characteristics of his hands. I would be grocery shopping in the produce aisle diagnosing the woman examining the apples with Cushing's syndrome by the shape of her face and the protuberance between her shoulders. Everywhere I turned it was new diagnosis on a topic matter I had just learned about. You just can't help it. Your eyes will be opened and the way you see the world is forever changed.

7.   BOARD PREP

By the time you finish your PA program, you will be well versed in taking tests. In fact, you may even be sick of taking tests. But one thing is for sure. You cannot enter the work force until you have passed the big one: the national boards. Although it may seem on your first day that they are so far away, please don't start school with that mindset. The weeks fly by and before you know it you will be enrolling in a prep course to pass your boards. The easiest way to tackle preparing for the big test is to start early. I highly recommend you study for each test as if you were about to take that portion of your boards. For instance, if you have a cardiology test, study as if you are taking the cardiology portion. At the time I am writing this the board questions are not lumped into particular sections but instead are given in a random order. Study for them anyway. There is no better time to prepare than while you are in school.

8.   THE STUFF THEY DON'T TELL YOU

The workload doesn't get easier but handling it does. The first few weeks and tests are always the scariest. You don't know what to expect. You don't know how you're going to do compared to your classmates. But soon after you start to get the feel for how we word our questions or what study techniques work best for you and you start to soar. It is not looked down upon to ask a question. In fact, it shows that you are listening and focused in on the subject matter. Likely someone else in the room has the same one you do, so don't ever feel alone. Finally, it is not the end of the world to miss a class or two and copy someone's notes, but don't make it a habit. This isn't college and it is hard to catch up if you miss multiple classes. Plus, at the end of the day, people's lives are in your hands so please take class seriously.

9.   WELCOME TO YOUR ONLY JOB

The first day of orientation our Program Director made a point to emphasize how time-consuming PA school is and how important it is to dedicate all of our attention to our school work. As you probably know, PA school is one of the few programs that does not give you the option to obtain the degree by attending school on a part time basis. It is full time or bust. My recommendation would be to treat school as though you have two full time jobs: one being going to school and the second being studying when you are home. I had two fellow students keep their part time jobs at local pharmacies because they thought it would make school easier. Both failed out before the second semester. If you are in PA school, welcome to your only job.

10.   ENJOY IT WHILE IT LASTS

So far, I have told you that PA school is a ton of hard work, the equivalent to two full time jobs, and is nothing like college so don't skip class. Now I get to tell you to enjoy it! This small amount of time is sacred. It is going to go by faster than you think. Do not take for granted that you have an entire team of medical staff members helping you become successful. Write thank you notes at the end of your rotations. Bring in cookies to show your appreciation. Let the staff know that you value their knowledge and are thankful they are willing to put in the work to pass it on to you. It will mean the world to them. Make as many good impressions as you can during your time at each rotation because of those good impressions may just lead to a job offer. And enjoy every single rotation. Because once you're in the real world, you can't go back.

11.   FROM CLASSMATES TO COLLEAGUES

Remember that you are all in this together. At the end of graduation, you (hopefully) will all pass your boards and enter the real world together. That is a big step that no one will understand like the ones taking that step with you. Make lasting friendships during your school years together. Find a group of core friends that have the same study habits as you and don't let them go. You will find that when you are in the real world and have a question about a topic pertaining to their particular specialty, it is really nice to have someone you trust to call. Or when you have had a stressful day or find yourself in the middle of a pandemic, a familiar voice on the other side of the phone fighting that battle with you is just what the PA ordered.

12.   THE LOVE HATE RELATIONSHIP

We all have these. The classes we love and the classes we hate. The topics we can read about for hours on end as if we are flipping through US Weekly Magazine and the topics that are painful to read even a paragraph in our textbook. The good news is at the end of school we get to choose our specialty. It doesn't get assigned to us (thank you Jesus!). You will know pretty quickly in didactic year which subject matter falls into which category for you. And you may not like me very much for saying this, but you need to treat them all with the same respect. You need to give as much attention, if not more, to the classes you hate as you do to the classes you love. In the real world, you don't get to pick which co-morbidities your patient has or which medical issues you want to skirt around. The things you studied just to get by will rear their ugly head and you will have to learn about it either way.

13.   DIARRHEA OF THE MOUTH

So, you spend all this time during didactic year studying your heart out and memorizing as much as you can in order to pass the upcoming test (and hopefully one day the boards). Then you move on to the next topic, rinse and repeat. You don't know how you are doing it. You're not sure where the information is being stored inside your head or if you're going to remember a lick of it after the test. But you keep doing this over and over and over until one day didactic year is done. Bring on the clinical year! You're sitting around the table with a practitioner and other students and someone asks you a question and out of nowhere the answer comes out. I sometimes call it divine intervention. Others call it diarrhea of the mouth. But take heart. Either way, what you spent so much time and effort memorizing the year before, you will out of nowhere recall it. Not all of it and not all the time, but more than you think you will. Just remember from tip #2 that you get what you put in. It is worth the time to memorize it early on and not when you are in the hot seat.

14. THE DOWNSIDE OF AN EMPTY STOMACH

Have you ever had that embarrassing experience where you had heard about it happening to other people but you didn't think it would ever happen to you? I mean you're smart, you over prepare for everything, and you know your body better than anyone. My very first rotation was in obstetrics and gynecology at a hospital in Westchester county. The surgeon and I got along so great that he invited me into the operating room (OR) with him to assist with a surgery. While we were in the OR lounge, he had a snack that I declined because I wasn't hungry and didn't want to look like I was scrounging for his food. Fast forward 30 minutes and I am sitting on the cold ground in the OR, fully scrubbed in with a sweet circulator nurse fanning me. Hypoglycemia had gotten the best of me. It is my non-negotiable rule for any students who scrub with me to this day that I am passing along to you. Even if you are not hungry, eat before the OR. Always.

15.   PRACTICE MAKES PERFECT

Of all the classes we take in PA school, any class that includes hands-on lessons is my favorite. It made me feel like we were in the thick of things, like we were actually grown up practitioners and we were going to save that mannequins' life. A little dramatic, I know. But I love those types of classes. It is the closest thing to the real-world experience in our didactic year that we get. The minute you learn to suture, practice when you get home. Buy oranges, bananas, pig's feet, chicken thighs, or the fake skin pads and practice, practice, practice. Practice everything from your sterile technique to the spacing of your sutures. And don't forget your ties. Learn a surgeon's knot, a two-handed tie and work your way to a one-handed tie. It is surgical etiquette to always start with a two-handed tie when in the OR. After a few times in the OR with the same surgeon and if you feel comfortable with the two-handed tie, you can ask if you can switch to a one-handed tie and show off that you've been practicing.

16.   SWEET DREAMS

Sleep when you can. I can almost stop this paragraph there with a microphone drop. Your body and mind are working non-stop during PA school. Don't be surprised if while your body needs more sleep, it is also hard to get good quality sleep. Try the best you can. You are no help to anyone (including yourself) if you're exhausted. Put the books away, turn the TV off, drop the phone and get some decent sleep. It will do your body good.

17.   RELIEF IS COMING

Sometimes it feels like the cycle is never ending. Sleep, Class, Study, Eat, Repeat. And every once in a while, there is no sleep because you have an all-night cram session for a big test the next morning. If you are ever exhausted or at your wit's end, I want you to dog ear the corner of this book or take a screen shot of it and read it as many times as you need. It will get better. This is not forever. This will pay off in the end. You will remember more than you think you will. You are here for a reason. It will get easier.

There is an end in sight. Relief is coming. Don't throw in the towel. You can do this.

18. THOSE WHO HAVE EARS LET THEM HEAR

Listening is one of the most important skills to have in medicine. I have diagnosed most of my patients not based on their physical exam or from their imaging, but from just their history alone. What is your patient telling you? It is important to master the skill of listening to what your patient is saying during their visit. What is your patient not telling you? Clarifying questions are a beautiful thing, but only if we ask them correctly. Ask open ended questions that allow them to describe their pain or ailment in their own words such as "when is your pain the worst?" Avoid leading questions as much as you can such as "would you say your pain is worse right before bed?" Sometimes the patient will answer how they think you want them to answer just to please you. Now back to the physical exam and imaging. Both are necessary and great ways to confirm your diagnosis (operative word: confirm). But if you are relying on them alone, you need to strengthen your history taking skills. One extra tip: if you live in an area that heavily speaks another language, I would highly recommend you learn how to perform a history and physical in that language. My PA program included a Spanish Medical course as a requirement to graduate and I still use those skills today.

19. YOU ARE GOING TO HAVE A GOOD DAY

This may sound like the corniest title ever. You may even be tempted to skip over this tip and move on to the next. But if you would, indulge me. You are what you think. You are what you put your focus on. And I am not going to sit here and tell you that you are going to have only good days from here on out. I mean who does that? But I am going to tell you that you're going to start your day telling yourself that. Get up from bed and tell yourself "I'm going to have a good day". You won't hit the mark every day but you will hit it more often than not by declaring it. And for those extremely rough days, before you go to bed stop and find the good. Maybe you learned a new fact today, maybe you mastered your surgical knots, or maybe you did nothing more than make it through one more day of school. Learn to find the good and celebrate it. This is a habit I highly recommend you continue throughout your entire career because the rough days don't stop. But, thank God, either do the good ones.

20. THE AMOUNT OF WORK IS EQUAL TO THE AMOUNT OF REWARD

Becoming a PA is one of the most rewarding jobs out there. And if you have read the tips above, you know that I have made it clear that this is not an easy road that we are on. We have put our blood, sweat and tears into studying hard, passing our boards, and finding jobs in the real world. The amount of work was intense. Thankfully, so is the reward. As Physician Assistants we have been given the opportunity and authority to positively impact every patient, even to the extreme point of saving a life. For that reason alone, the benefit of the rewards will always far outweigh the stress and sacrifices we made to get here. Hold on to that tightly. It will get you through the roughest of times.

THE NEW PA

21. INTENTIONALLY DO GOOD

One of the first things they teach you in medicine is that by the time you are done you will have the knowledge base to heal your patient. Our course of actions will determine the patient's outcome. When I am invited to speak at a PA school orientation, to teach a class for the first time or to address a graduating class, I always use the same opening remark. "Every time you touch a patient you can harm a patient. Every. Time. There is no in-between." I have seen patients become gravely ill from an urinary tract infection after a very simple foley catheter placement. I have seen a patient bleed out in the ICU from a practitioner packing their abdominal wound too forcefully. I have seen a patient going into a severe allergic reaction because the practitioner didn't check their allergy list before placing a medication order. We never intend to harm our patients. But we need to be mindful that complications are real and some even lethal. It is our job to be careful and intentional to do no harm.

22.   THE ULTIMATE GIFT

Of all the things we will accomplish during our training and our careers, bringing life into this world is one of the best gifts we can give our patients. Watching a baby take their first breath while their mother's face turns from exhausted to ecstatic is one of the most precious moments this career has to offer. It is one of those few times that deserves a brief pause to soak it all in. We had a part in this and it is beautiful. As Physician Assistants we have been blessed with the opportunity to take part in the ultimate gift: life. Not just bringing life into this world, but the ability to save lives. Never take this for granted. And please know in the deepest part of your heart that no matter what field you choose, you have the responsibility to save a life. Whether it is in a dermatology office diagnosing skin cancer or in a radiology suite taken a second look at the brain MRI because something just doesn't feel right. The ability to save a life is not isolated for just one field of medicine. This gift is for us all.

23. BE FLEXIBLE

One of the best things about choosing to become a Physician Assistant is the flexibility within the fields of medicine. We have been given the gift of being able to switch specialties without having to go back to school or completing additional residencies. In other words, you're not stuck. Keep an open mind during all of your rotations before choosing which one is right for you. There may be more than one specialty that catches your eye. For those that do, make sure that you find a way to keep in touch with key players in that field. Ask for their email or save their cell phone number. This will come in handy when you are applying for a job and need a letter of recommendation. I highly recommend if you are using a preceptor that you read the student evaluation form that they completed for you prior to asking them to write a letter of recommendation. And always put your best foot forward.   As preceptors we are always looking for potential employees.

24.   SURGERY VS MEDICINE WARS

You may be one of those people who entered PA school already knowing the specific medical field you wanted to enter. Or maybe you were one of those students who graduated, realized there are several specialties you enjoy and still have no idea which way to go. I have found that most of us find our way somewhere in the middle. No matter when you discover your calling, I want to share a piece of advice with you. In most cases you are either medical or you are surgical. But either way you need to learn to respect the other. This is one of those lessons you are going to want to learn early. Do not buy into the hype that one is better than the other or that there is this need to continue medical versus surgical wars. When it comes down to it, one cannot exist without the other. We are all in this together with the same main goal, to enhance the patient's life.

25. CAPTURE THE MOMENT

One of the best decisions I made early on in my career was to save a memento from the major moments that happened at work. Something tangible that would serve as a reminder of the event that just took place. My very first job as a Physician Assistant was in the newborn intensive care unit. It was at a community hospital right up the street from a larger, well known hospital. And although we did not have a large amount of extremely premature babies in our unit on a regular basis, I will never forget the morning that we did. I was in practice for several months at this point and a mother presented in premature labor at 28 weeks gestation. When the baby was born, we did everything we could to keep her alive and we were successful. I left work that day with my first memento, a diaper that could fit in the palm of my hand. It was given to me from the package of diapers we had opened when the baby was born. I keep it with my other mementos, each one with a different meaning to me. The diaper serves a reminder that miracles can happen every day and sometimes we are blessed enough to take part in them.

26. BRAG BOOKS ARE NOT JUST FOR REPS

The first time I had ever heard of a brag book I was at a friendly dinner with few wound care reps. The newest member of the team was pitching a product to me that would help my surgical patients. During the pitch, he made sure to mention his most recent accomplishment when his boss and my friend quickly chimed in. "Make sure to put that in your brag book". I'm sorry, what? A brag book? Is this a real thing? I was educated on more than just their products that night. My friend went on to inform me that most reps have a brag book, a book of all of their achievements and bragging rights. They use this as a resource to prep for pitches or interviews with potential clients. What a great idea and something that is not job specific. I started to share the news with other practitioners about the value of a brag book. This is something I recommend you start early and reference prior to any job interviews and while building your resume. Please know that this is not meant to make you walk around with a puffed-out chest. It is simply a means of reminding you of your strengths and accomplishments so you enter the interview prepared.

27. WHAT YOU DON'T KNOW

One of the scariest subsets of practitioners to me is those who don't know what they don't know. Let me say that again. We all are relatively aware of our strengths and our weaknesses. If you are one of the few that is not aware, don't worry. Your first job will make it pretty clear for you. But there is this portion of all of us who think we know how to do something correctly, when in actuality we really don't. Because we think we are doing it right, we don't realize that we actually don't know what it is that we think we know. So, we just keep doing it. It is our duty to make sure that we are trained for our specialty and to stay up to date on treatment plans. When starting a new job, no matter how many years of experience you have, please make sure that there is a document signed by your manager that states you have been observed and are free to perform your duties independently. This will legally protect you and show that you actually do know what you're doing! It is also the time to be honest about what you don't know.

28. IT'S COMPLICATED

Before becoming a PA, when someone said M&M my mind immediately went to the candy. After more than a decade of a career in surgery, now when someone says M&M my mind immediately goes to our Morbidity and Mortality conference. While I was working for one of the more well-known health care systems, M&M was seen as a firing squad. A practitioner or surgical resident would present a patient along with their complication and the surgeons in the room would rapidly fire difficult questions and voice their concerns. The person behind the podium, whether they were involved in the case or not, owned that patient and their complication. It was their job to explain or defend the actions made that resulted in the complication. Although it may sound horrible, it is meant for educational purposes. The goal was to walk out of that room with a deep understanding of what went wrong so that no one would make that mistake again. To humbly understand that just because it did not happen to you, does not mean that it could never happen to you. Complications are a risk we take in this profession. It is part of our duty to learn from these complications, whether ours or our colleagues, to protect our patients as much as possible.

29. NEVER ENDING LEARNING

One of the many beautiful things about a career in medicine is that we are constantly moving forward. With the continual creation of new devices, new medications and new vaccines, the innovative world of medicine is captivating. And it is part of our job to keep up with it all. Now, you don't have to be well versed in every area of medicine. But the learning doesn't end just because we left the classroom. Make sure that you keep on top of your journal reading, logging your CMEs and attending conferences that will push you to learn more. If you have mastered reading x-rays, move on to courses where you learn how to use the ultrasound and read the sonograms. We work in a field that allows an old dog to learn new tricks. Take full advantage of it. You never know where your skills will take you. And in the words of my father, Richard Bubbico, they can take a lot from you, but they can never take your education. Become as educated as possible.

30.   COCKY PEOPLE

Somewhere in between starting my career and precepting PA students I came up with the line "cocky people kill people". I found that it didn't matter if you were new or experienced, a student or already held your board certification. If you acted like you knew it all, it became apparent to me that you were likely at a higher risk of harming a patient. I have noticed that these practitioners are less likely to ask for help, more likely to assume they know the diagnosis and treatment plan and have a hard time getting out of their own way. Plus, a handful of them will read this paragraph and not even realize they are one of them! Now, there are plenty of very well-educated people out there who have a low complication rate. So obviously this statement of cocky people is more to keep you grounded and less to be statistically analyzed. Be humble, be aware that you may not know it all, and be willing to ask for help.

31. DELIVERING BAD NEWS

This is one of the harder parts of the job. I wanted to include a couple of tips that I have picked up along the way in hopes that it will make this difficult moment for you a bit smoother. Always use the name of the patient. Whether you are telling a son their mother just passed or you are telling a woman she has breast cancer. The patient needs to know that they are known to you and are not just another patient we check off of a list. Sit down when telling them. Never stand over them. This is a sensitive matter and they need to know you're not going to run away. By sitting with them it makes them feel like you are with them and they have your attention. Apologizing for the situation and letting them know you are there for them should always go hand in hand. This is a scary time for the patient and they need to be reminded you are on their side. Listen patiently to their questions or their outburst of anger and make sure they have someone with them who can help absorb the information that may be missed in the shock of it all. Although it is never easy to deliver bad news, this is one of the parts that gets easier with time and experience.

32. YOUR FIRST LOSS

I will never forget his name. Because of HIPAA I cannot state it here but know that it is in my heart forever. I was on my medicine rotation (as a surgery girl this was a hard rotation to muster through), when my best friend and I were asked to collect a blood culture from a patient who was not doing well. He was elderly and near the end of his life. The family had made the decision to make him comfort measures only and our attending on call wanted to see what was causing this sepsis. We went in to draw the blood and our hearts sank. Although he did not open his eyes or acknowledge our presence, we hoped he could hear us as we spoke gently to him as we explained why we were there. Within a few minutes, we recognized that his breathing had become agonal. The end was near. My friend stopped attempting to draw the blood, held his hand, called him by name and let him know we were here and it was okay. The man died with us holding his hands. The first patient you lose will always stay with you. Their name, how it happened, how you felt. All of it. Take time to process the loss and to ask for help when needed. Do not carry that burden alone.

33.   YOUR FIRST SAVE

The first patient I saved was a 40-week full term baby that had a cord wrapped around his neck and a mother that was struggling to naturally deliver the baby. He was fully formed, otherwise healthy baby except by the time he was delivered and handed to me he was entirely blue. He was not breathing and for the first time in my career I felt entirely alone with the weight of the world on my shoulders. It is okay to feel that stress, but it is not okay to let that stress take over. I shook it off and did was I was trained to do. We saved the baby that day. Saving a life leaves you with this feeling of exhilaration that is unlike anything else. Take a moment, find that memento, and be thankful that we get to play a part in this.

34.   ASSOCIATIONS AND BEYOND

So, remember how I was saying that it is important to make sure we always keep learning to stay up to date with the ever-changing times of medicine (or did you skip over #29)? One of the easiest ways to stay on top of learning, finding good conferences and even job hunting is to join associations. The American

Academy of Physician Assistants, AAPA, is a great place to start. The AAPA will send out email blasts with great CME articles and will keep you up to date with other changes going on within our profession. The educational conferences will allow you to branch out and make friends within your specialty. They offer great resources and educational materials during the conference such as hand on classes for anyone who needs to sharpen their skillset. I strongly recommend that you sign up for an additional association that is directly related to your specialty. The generic CME articles will help you pass your boards, while the specialty associations will help you take better care of your patients. Either way, both are extremely beneficial.

35.   CAUGHT UP IN THE CHAOS

It is so easy to get caught up in the chaos of it all. Whether it is a jam-packed day in the office, back to back trauma consults in the emergency department or a marathon of surgeries, it is easy to get lost in the hustle and bustle. Sometimes, this turns into feeling like you're on auto-pilot just trying to make it through another exhausting day. It gets easier. Don't give up.

Remember to breathe, especially during a code. Stay calm. Remember what you were taught. Start from the top and work your way down the list. Airway. Breathing. Circulation. You were trained for this. You know what you're doing. Don't let the stress weigh you down. When all is said and done, stop what you're doing and take a moment to let it all go. We are all super proud of you.

36. NEGOTIATIONS

Negotiating as a new Physician Assistant can feel like you are stuck with your back up against the wall. You do not have any experience, your skill set is far from perfected, and your base salary is $0. So how can you make sure that you're getting a fair deal? You will need to do your homework. Research the salary of Physician Assistants in that area or state for the specific job that you are being offered. Find out about your benefits. Specifically, what type of health, dental and eye insurance you will receive and what type of retirement plan do they offer (aka what options do you have as to where to invest your money). Ask about paid time off, sick time and CME time. Each job should provide you with a separate amount of time off that does not come from your PTO bank and a set amount of money to be used towards furthering your education that does not come out of your salary. And finally, ask about overtime. Even if you are salary based, if you need to come in on a weekend or holiday, will you get paid? It is best to have all of the information so that you can make an educated decision.

37. ONE NEGATIVE ENCOUNTER

If you haven't heard yet, patients that stays in the hospital will likely receive a survey sometime after discharge. These survey results are then reported back to the hospital so that we can evaluate the feedback and make changes as needed. This overall feedback is taken very seriously by administration, and has been known to be attached to employee's bonuses. If you work in the outpatient setting, you're not spared. Although the patient may not receive a national survey, we can't forget the power of negative reviews on the internet or the negative posts on social media. We must be mindful that one negative encounter can ruin their whole experience. The art of service recovery is extremely helpful in this area.

Ask the patient how their experience was and what you can do to make it better. Make sure they feel heard and valued. Do not get defensive but instead welcome constructive criticism. Thank them for the positive or negative feedback. We can always learn from both.

38. CODING

This is one of those things that they do not teach you about in PA school but has a massive impact on you in the real world. Coding and billing are much more of a science than an art. You have the potential to make money every time you see a patient. Whether it is a well visit, assisting in the operating room, a consult, placing a splint on a broken extremity, performing a procedure, and the list goes on and on. I would strongly recommend that you write down the most popular codes that you will be using (you can ask your colleagues or your boss on what those may be) and keep them handy. Eventually you will likely memorize them, but know these bills are usually monitored closely to make sure they were placed and that the revenue was received. It is a great idea to get a head start in this area. Anything you forget to bill for is lost revenue for your employer. Make sure that you stay up to date with the laws and regulations regarding billing.

39. CONSULTS

The best way to call a consult is prepared. There are so many times in the beginning of my career where I could call a consult only to be met with what felt like one hundred questions that I had no answer to. That equals one hundred opportunities for me to realize that I was ill prepared to call this consult. My biggest piece of advice to you is when you are calling a consult have the full picture in front of you. That includes the lab results, the imaging, all of the progress notes (yes even from other services), and for the love of God please see the patient. Being on the other end now, the worst is when I ask a question about the physical state of the patient and the practitioner tells me they don't know because they didn't examine the patient. Don't be that person. And don't fret if you forget things the first few times you call a consult. This gets easier with experience. If you can, get ahead of the other person on the line by presenting the patient in a succinct manner with all the pertinent details. My opening line always includes three things: the age, gender and probable diagnosis. This helps the person I am calling follow along with my thought process as I reveal the other pertinent information and has saved me a ton of time!

THE EXPERIENCED PA

40. YOU'RE NOT STUCK

One of the beautiful things about being a PA is the flexibility. Not just switching from one field to the other without having to sit for your boards or go back to attend a residency, but that we don't have to stay in the clinical world forever. We can take a leadership position and still work in the healthcare system at an administrative level. We can take our years of experience and become a professor at PA school or we can teach classes such as anatomy and physiology for those students in the undergraduate level. We can completely switch gears and work for pharmaceutical or medical device companies or we can enter the field of legal medicine and review insurance cases. The world is our oyster and from one experienced PA to another, you're not stuck.

41.   IT'S NOT A COMPETITION

If you haven't learned this yet, learn it now. This is one of the most important tips in this book. You are not in a competition. Not with your colleagues, not with other departments, not with those above you, and not with those below you. Your knowledge is a God given gift that is to be used to heal the sick. It is not a weapon to be used against others or to boast about how much you know. Sometime when we get caught up in it all we tend to forget this. We try to prove our point to our colleagues, the patients or ourselves in a way that comes off aggressive. You're an experienced PA. You know what you know and you know what you don't. Be a light to those who need your expertise and ask for help when you need theirs. Do not let pride stand between you and your patient care.

42. HEALTHY HABITS

We have chosen an insanely rewarding field that also comes with its baggage of stress and chaos. It is important to find a way a healthy way to unwind and let the stress of the day go. I remember at my PA school interview they asked how I handle stress and what I do to unwind. I told them I have the healthy habits of an 80-year-old woman. I knit, crochet and do needlepoint to unwind. Some days I hit the gym harder than my non-stressful days. Other days I just sit. No noise, no distractions, just 5 minutes of nothing but sitting. It is so important that we create healthy habits that help us unwind because at the end of the day burnout is real. My other strong recommendation that I encourage every person to do is to find a therapist and have them on retainer. Find them early (before you are in the thick of the mess). Meet with them a few times a year, or more if needed, to evaluate how you're handling it all. There is no shame in speaking with a professional. Ever.

43. THE HONEST LEADER

One of the best gifts we can give others is honest feedback. Whether it is our direct reports, our students, or even our leaders, it is important to be deliberate and honest. Telling a student or employee they're doing okay when they actually have weak spots that need work is an injustice not only to them but also to our profession. Now, please take a moment to recognize what I am saying. There is a big difference between disrespectfully honest and deliberately honest. First, one can get you fired while the other can actually result in a positive change. Second, one makes you look like a crappy leader while the other shows that you are fair and approachable. Part of leadership is having to address the issues head on. But it does not mean that we have to be aggressive with how we handle the issue. Be deliberate about what you say and how you say it. We then in turn are more likely to get honest feedback back.

44. THE POWER OF GIVING BACK

By this point in our career, we are bursting at the seams with knowledge and experience. We have put in the blood, sweat and tears to get here. We had to make a lot of sacrifices along the way. It has finally paid off and now it is time to give back. Whether it is teaching a class, precepting students on their clinical rotations, or spending time speaking to a friend of a friend's daughter who is considering PA school, it is so important that we give back to the profession we poured our hearts into. We get to have a part in building strong PA's that will take over for us and lead the way by passing along our knowledge. In the words of the great T.D. Jakes "success is not success without a successor". We can build these wildly successful careers, but if we have no one to pass the baton to when we walk away, can we really consider it a success?

45. THE WEAKNESS IN US ALL

Every year of being in practice is a year that we get stronger. Stronger in our skill sets, stronger in our knowledge base and stronger in appearing like we have got this thing mastered. Sometimes, we ride the strong train for so long we forget that we still have weak spots. These areas of weakness that over the years have been overshadowed by our strengths that we forget they even exist. This is your invitation to re-examine your practices, your skillsets, and your knowledge base to see where your area of weakness lies. You get to choose whether or not this is an area that you would like to work on to make a strength. But my ask is that even if you do nothing about it, at the very minimum acknowledge that you have them. Put a name to the weakness so that when it rears its head, you will know to pass the buck or strengthen up.

46. PRACTICE WHAT YOU PREACH

I cannot tell you how many times I have preached on preventative health. "Did you get your colonoscopy? I'm sorry, how long has it been since you've had an annual physical exam? I don't think we can list your gynecologist as your PCP in your chart ma'am. And while we're on the topic don't forget your mammogram." It is so important for our patients to keep up with routine monitoring to prevent or to have early detection of any illnesses. But when is the last time we went to the doctor? When is the last time we actually made the call to set up an appointment instead of calling a colleague to curb side them for advice? If you already have your preventive appointments, you can skip to the next bullet point. But for those of you that don't, I want to push you to pick up the phone and make the appointment. It might just save your life.

47. YOU'RE IN IT TO WIN IT

I wish I could sit down with you and discuss how long you've been in the business, hear all of your amazing stories about your experiences, and find out what your plans are for your future. Would you do it all over again? Would you recommend this profession to someone else? Did this turn out to be what you expected? There have been a few times where I have thought of throwing in the towel. And in case you are ever there, I wanted to include this section as a reminder to never give up. You are in this profession for a reason. I like to tell myself that I may just be here to save someone's life who I haven't even met yet, that I still have work to do, and that I could meet someone on this path that will completely change my life. I'm with you and happy to stand shoulder to shoulder in this profession.

48. PTO IS SACRED

Did you know the sabbath was meant to not just be a time of rest but a time to enjoy God's creations and draw close to him? My medical rotation was at a Jewish hospital in the Bronx. The first Friday I was there I stepped on the elevator to go home and noticed that every single button was pushed. I remember thinking to myself this is like that scene from Elf where Will Ferrell gets excited can't help himself so he pushes all the elevator buttons just to see them light up. I was later educated that it was to honor the Sabbath. If the buttons were pushed for us, we would not have to do the work of pushing them. A time of rest is considered is truly sacred in the Jewish and Christian faith. And it got me thinking. If the times of rest are sacred, we need to take them more often. I have started a tradition where every season I take one week off. Even if I have nowhere to go. This sacred paid time off (PTO) is a time for me to rest and reset, to enjoy life and to step away from it all. It has been life changing and I invite you to do the same.

49. FURTHERING YOUR DEGREE

By the time I started my second job as a Physician Assistant I had three science degrees. Several months after starting this position I was asked to help take charge of a service line that needed to be revamped. To be honest, it was not my first choice but I jumped on the opportunity in hopes that it would help further my career. I ended up really enjoying the service and it caught the attention of our department chairman. He sat me down in his office and said I want you to go back to school. That was the last thing I wanted to hear. I had not been out of PA school for that long so the toll of being a student was still fresh in my mind. I'm not sure I wanted to go back to school. Ever. But I prayed about it and felt that it was the direction God was leading me in, so I applied to a local MBA program. Furthering my degree was one of the best decisions I have ever made. This degree has allowed me to speak the same language as our board of directors, to catch the attention of the executive leaders and to be promoted multiple times. If you are considering furthering your education in any way, I want you to know I am cheering you on. It has the potential to change your life forever.

50.   KEEP THE FAITH

This is a long road full of twists and turns, ups and downs, things you didn't see coming and things you saw coming from a mile away. It's not always easy, and sometimes it feels like it is not always worth it. But take heart, for he has overcome the world3. You are never alone. Keep the faith when things are good, when things are bad, and when things are in between. Don't lose your hope. Love when you want to hate. Pray when you want to complain. Thank Him for every good thing when you want to throw in the towel and walk away. He created you with a purpose. I don't know how long we have in this profession, but I do know this. God is good. And we should continue to do His will as long as we have breath in our lungs. He has given us a talent to treat patients and be a part of their healing process. I can't think of a better gift to be shared with others.

OTHER RESOURCES:

Jakes, T. [Bishop T.D. Jakes]. (2017, July 11).
Success is not a Success without a Successor.
[Tweet]. Retrieved from
https://twitter.com/bishopjakes/status/8848196391125
27873?lang=en

Revelations 2:17

John 16:33

READ OTHER

50 THINGS TO KNOW

BOOKS

50 Things to Know

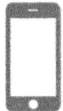

Stay up to date with new releases on Amazon:
https://amzn.to/2VPNGr7

Mailing List: Join the 50 Things to Know
Mailing List to Learn About New Releases

50 Things to Know

Please leave your honest review of this book on Amazon and Goodreads. We appreciate your positive and constructive feedback. Thank you.